Frequently Asked Questions

all about
st. john's wort

HYLA CASS, MD

AVERY PUBLISHING GROUP

Garden City Park • New York

The information contained in this book is based upon the research and personal and professional experiences of the author. They are not intended as a substitute for consulting with your physician or other health care provider. Any attempt to diagnose and treat an illness should be done under the direction of a health care professional.

The publisher does not advocate the use of any particular health care protocol, but believes the information in this book should be available to the public. The publisher and author are not responsible for any adverse effects or consequences resulting from the use of any of the suggestions, preparations, or procedures discussed in this book. Should the reader have any questions concerning the appropriateness of any procedure or preparation mentioned, the author and the publisher strongly suggest consulting a professional health care advisor.

ISBN: 0-89529-893-7

Printed in the United States of America

10   9   8   7   6   5   4   3

Contents

Introduction

Feeling depressed? Overwhelmed by sadness and a lack of hope? St. John's wort, a time-cherished medicinal herb, can likely help.

The benefits of St. John's wort may be subtle in some people, such as Laurie, a twenty-seven-year-old secretary. "St. John's wort is a wonderful cure for the blues," she related. "Its effects are barely noticeable until you realize that the things that used to aggravate you no longer affect you the way they once did."

Other people have much more dramatic recoveries from depression. Kara, a thirty-five-year-old store clerk, used St. John's wort and said, "I feel alert, am in a good mood, and feel like doing things. I really like it!"

Jack, a forty-year-old playwright, was also appreciative of this traditional folk medicine. "St. John's wort has saved my life and has given me a new look at life," he explained.

Likewise for Marcia. "I was on Prozac for two years and just about went broke buying it, not to mention the side effects!" exclaimed the twenty-four-year-old graduate student. "Then I switched to St. John's wort, and I feel more alert and less tired, with no side effects at all! All in all, I think it's great."

These are true, if amazing, personal stories, and thousands of people have shared similar experiences. So it's no surprise that St. John's wort has been the subject of headlines in major newspapers, magazines, medical journals, and other media around the world including *Newsweek, The New York Times, USA Today,* and the television show *20/20.*

For the more than 18 million people in the United States who suffer from depression, St. John's wort may be the answer to their prayers. Why? Because research has shown that this humble herb with yellow flowers has all the benefits of prescription antidepressants such as Prozac and Zoloft, but without the side effects and at one-tenth the cost. In fact, in recent years, St. John's wort has been the treatment of choice in Europe, outnumbering Prozac in purchases by twenty to one. And just recently, a $4.3-million federally funded large-scale study was launched in the United States to test its effectiveness in the treatment of depression.

You may be wondering how a simple herb can possibly be as effective as a patented prescription medication. In fact, St. John's wort is not only as good as prescription medications, but in many cases it is actually more effective and certainly safer. Furthermore, it has many other beneficial effects, easing anxiety, premenstrual syndrome (PMS), and insomnia. St. John's wort also contains natural antiviral and anti-inflammatory compounds.

As more and more people take charge of their own health and well-being, the need is rising for authoritative and yet understandable resources to help cut through the often confusing information. In *All About St. John's Wort*, I have drawn on my many years of clinical practice of integrative (or "natural") psychiatry, which has included success-fully prescribing St. John's wort for many patients. This book is also supported by the latest medical and scientific research, so you can read the most accurate and up-to-date information on this remarkable herb. Much of this information will be illustrated by the comments of real people— patients, associates, and others who have used and benefited from St. John's wort.

In the following pages, you will learn all about the signs and symptoms of depression. You will also learn:

• How St. John's wort safely and effectively corrects depression.
• How it is used to treat anxiety, PMS, and insomnia.

- About its recommended dosages.
- About its side effects.
- How it compares with antidepressant medications.
- About the forms it comes in.
- About the scientific research that supports its use.
- About other natural remedies and lifestyle choices that counter depression.

Life is precious, and it is to be enjoyed fully. While occasional periods of sadness and feeling down are to be expected and normal, you don't want these feelings to prevent you from having a satisfying and rewarding life. St. John's wort, as you'll find, can help keep you on track.

1.

Test Yourself—Are You Depressed?

Think you're depressed? Or just temporarily feeling down? To find out if you're depressed and need professional help, take this quick quiz.

Here's how to do it: For each question, circle the answer that comes closest to describing the way you feel. Circle "1" if you don't feel that way at all or if you feel that way only a part of the time. Circle "2" if you feel that way some of the time. Circle "3" if you feel that way much of the time. Circle "4" if you feel that way most or all of the time. (If you don't want to mark up this book, just write down the numbers on a separate sheet of paper.) Answer the questions honestly.

1. I feel downhearted, blue, and sad.

    1   2   3   4

2. I feel worse in the morning.

    1   2   3   4

3. I have crying spells, or feel like it.

    1   2   3   4

4. I have trouble sleeping through the night.

    1   2   3   4

5. My appetite is poor.

    1   2   3   4

6. I feel unattractive and not likable.

    1   2   3   4

7. I am losing weight without trying.

    1   2   3   4

8. I prefer to be alone.

    1   2   3   4

9. I feel fearful.

    1   2   3   4

10. I feel tired.

    1   2   3   4

11. I have trouble concentrating.

    1   2   3   4

12. It is an effort to do the things I used to do.

    1   2   3   4

13. I am restless and can't keep still.

    1   2   3   4

14. I feel hopeless about the future.

    1   2   3   4

15. I am irritable.

    1   2   3   4

16. I find it difficult to make decisions.

    1   2   3   4

17. I feel that I am not needed.

    1   2   3   4

18. My life feels empty and pointless.

    1   2   3   4

19. I feel that others would be better off if I were dead.

    1   2   3   4

20. I do not enjoy the things I used to enjoy.

    1   2   3   4

When you are finished, add up all of the circled numbers. If your score is:

Below 30, you are within the normal range.

Between 30 and 50, you are minimally to mildly depressed.

Over 50, you are moderately to seriously depressed.

If the quiz results indicate that you may be depressed, or if you are experiencing suicidal thoughts, speak to your physician or health-care practitioner to first rule out a physical cause for your problems. If necessary, your doctor should refer you to a psychiatrist, preferably one with an orthomolecular orientation—that is, a doctor who uses natural rather than synthetic substances whenever possible. Otherwise, in addition to a therapist, be sure to consult a naturopath or other natural-medicine practitioner to look for an underlying nutritional or biochemical imbalance.

2.

What Is St. John's Wort?

In this chapter, I will introduce you to the basics of St. John's wort—what it is, how it works, what you can expect from it, and when you should use it. I will describe the broad range of conditions that this amazing nonprescription herb can treat, including anxiety, depression, insomnia, PMS, menopausal symptoms, attention deficit disorder, and even burns and wounds when the herb is applied topically.

Q. What is St. John's wort?

A. St. John's wort, whose botanical name is *Hypericum perforatum*, is a bushy perennial plant with yellow flowers that commonly grows wild, but that, as a medicinal herb, is grown commercially. It is native to many parts of the world, including Europe, Asia, and the United States, especially the Pacific Northwest, where it is known as klamath weed. In fact, there were programs there to eradicate it as a pest plant until its newfound popularity changed its status.

Q. From where did St. John's wort get its unusual name?

A. The botanical name *Hypericum* comes from the Greek words *yper*, meaning "upper," and *eikon*, meaning "image." The Greeks and Romans believed that St. John's wort protected them from evil spirits and witches' spells, and often placed the herb in their homes and above statues of their gods. Perhaps the spirits and spells they feared were really depression and anxiety, mental disorders with no obvious physical causes.

The early Christians incorporated many ancient beliefs into their new religion. Pre-existing spring rituals, for instance, were renamed as saints' feast days. In this tradition, Christian mystics renamed *Hypericum perforatum* after St. John the Baptist. The herb was traditionally collected on St. John's Day, June 24, and soaked in olive oil for days to produce a blood-red anointing oil, said to symbolize the blood of the saint. "Wort" has nothing to do with skin warts. It's the Old English word for "plant."

Q. What can I expect from St. John's wort?

A. Consider the case of Kate, a forty-eight-year-old married author and public speaker, as fairly typical. Kate had a hectic lifestyle and said, "While on an impossible deadline, I had a total collapse. I was exhausted, stressed, and depressed. My doctor put me on Prozac, but it made me even more depressed, and then I couldn't sleep. He gave me sleeping pills that zonked me, and that was it. I stopped the Prozac. Then I read about St. John's wort, and tried it, 300 mg twice daily. I figured it couldn't hurt! Three weeks later, my husband Mike suddenly noticed: 'You're different! You seem more relaxed, less tense. What's going on?'"

Kate hadn't told her husband that she was taking St. John's wort, but her change in attitude was obvious. "One of the most dramatic things I began to notice is I felt happy and joyful in the morning. It was never like this on Prozac. I'm more energetic and focused, and there's more laughter!" Her good news continued. "Our sex life had always been sporadic and difficult. Since starting St. John's wort, however, we have had an extraordinary change for the better, and it has continued." In a separate conversation with me, Mike was even more effusive than Kate. "I can't believe how she's changed. She's always been so tense, barely available, especially when she's stressed. Now, she's a delight. We are having the time of our lives!"

Q. Is Kate's experience typical?

A. You might argue that this sounds too good to be true, that Kate's experience is an isolated incidence or that she was responding to the power of suggestion. According to the research I have read, reports from other physicians and practitioners, and my own clinical experience, Kate's is not an isolated case. Another woman reported, "St. John's wort changed my whole life, my outlook, everything. It's like a veil lifted from around my head. I've never felt so good. And I'm dreaming again, and remembering my dreams. I can hardly believe it!"

Q. How long has St. John's wort been used as a therapeutic herb?

A. The oldest records of its use are from Greek and Roman times, about two thousand years ago. Dioscorides, the foremost Greek herbalist, recommended it for sciatica and malaria, and as a diuretic and a female tonic. Pliny the Elder, the Roman naturalist, found it effective, when mixed with wine, against snakebite. Later, the Crusaders carried the plant to protect themselves from sorcery and also used the soaked flowers and leaves as an ointment to help heal the wounds of battle.

The first *London Pharmacopoeia*, published in 1618, recommended that the flowers be placed in oil and allowed to stand for three weeks. The resulting tincture could then be used for wounds and bruises. Other traditional folk uses for St. John's wort include the treatment of gout, rheumatism, and jaundice. Native Americans used it for diarrhea, fever, snakebite, and wounds and other skin problems. It later served as a valuable medicine for treating soldiers' wounds during the Civil War. St. John's wort was also prescribed by the homeopaths of the period for a variety of ailments, as it is to this day.

Q. Why hasn't St. John's wort been used in the United States until now?

A. While St. John's wort has been known to healers for thousands of years, it has only now become an "overnight sensation" in the modern media. Why is this? Toward the end of the nineteenth century, the medical establishment in the United States turned its back on traditional folk remedies. Teachings that had been passed down through the ages were dismissed as primitive superstitions.

Medical authorities lobbied Congress and the state legislatures for the prohibition of herbal medicine. Their goal was to produce pharmaceutical medications by isolating the plants' so-called active ingredients and discarding the rest. Now, of course, we realize these "extras" are often the secret to a plant's strength and healing power. Current laws still restrict making specific healing claims on herbal-medicine labels. On the other hand, in Europe—in Germany in particular—herbal medicine is part of medical-school curriculum, and doctor's prescribe St. John's wort on a regular basis.

Q. What is St. John's wort used for currently?

A. Research in treating patients with mild to moderately severe depression has shown that St. John's wort relieves the symptoms of sadness, helplessness, hopelessness, anxiety, headache, and exhaustion, and with minimal side effects. It is also useful in seasonal affective disorder and PMS, as an antiviral, and as an anti-inflammatory agent. The German Commission E, similar to the American Food and Drug Administration (FDA), has approved St. John's wort for two general categories of use. First, it can be taken orally for psychological disturbances, depressive states, sleep disorders, and anxiety, including that associated with menopause. As an oil taken orally, it is also approved for stomach and gastrointestinal complaints, since it has anti-diarrheal activity. Second, as an oil applied topically, it is approved for the treatment of wounds, bruises, muscle aches, and first-degree burns.

Q. What about using St. John's wort for stress?

A. Stress causes an imbalance in the chemicals that normally help the brain to function, leading to anxiety and depression. While St. John's wort won't take the stress away, it will help you to deal with it better. In the words of my patient Janice, "Before, I was stressed out and felt hopeless. Now that I'm in balance, even though I'm dealing with exactly the same issues, I feel like there is a light at the end of the tunnel."

Q. Does St. John's wort treat anxiety as well, and how does it do this?

A. Such prescription medications as Valium, Xanax, and Klonopin, called the benzodiazepines, exert their sedative actions through the calming neurotransmitter gamma-aminobutyric acid (GABA). St. John's wort has a high affinity for GABA receptors, which would explain its sedative and anti-anxiety effects. Newer research suggests that GABA may additionally be involved in antidepressant reactions.

Q. **I notice that I sleep much better when I take St. John's wort regularly, yet it doesn't make me drowsy during the day. Why is this?**

A. St. John's wort works with the body's own sleep-promoting mechanism to bring on restful sleep. Prescription sedatives, on the other hand, often produce grogginess, resulting in a hangover effect the next morning. They can also be addictive. Instead of drugging your brain into submission, St. John's wort enhances its natural actions, producing deep, restful sleep. Unlike most antidepressants, it does not interfere with rapid-eye-movement (REM) sleep, which is essential for mental health, since the subconscious mind busily analyzes the day's events and processes feelings during this time.

Since it can take a week or so for this effect to begin, St. John's wort is recommended mainly for recurring insomnia and not just an occasional restless night. It appears that St. John's wort enhances the effects of melatonin, a hormone that regulates our sleep and awake cycles. One study showed that a dose of 90 drops of St. John's wort tincture daily over a three-week period significantly increased nighttime melatonin levels.

Q. A friend of mine uses St. John's wort for panic attacks. Is this a common use?

A. I have had patients with panic disorder who would not leave home without it! Panic attacks can strike those with the disorder at any time, unrelated to external events. During a panic attack, you feel a sense of panic and impending doom that is terrifying, though it is not really dangerous. It just feels that way! Besides functioning as an antidepressant, St. John's wort is an excellent antianxiety agent. However, it must be taken regularly, at the ususal doses, and not just before stressful events, since it needs time to build up in the system to be most effective. During times of increased stress, you can also add kava, a Polynesian herb, at a dose of 70 mg or so of standardized extract (containing 30-percent kavalactones) three times daily.

Q. What about using St. John's wort for PMS?

A. PMS, or premenstrual syndrome, is a common disorder that afflicts many women about seven days prior to the onset of their menstrual period, with moodiness, irritability, bloating, and fatigue. Many women have reported that their usual PMS symptoms stopped after they began taking St. John's wort for depression. For centuries, herbalists have recognized the herb's value in treating the discomforts associated with the menstrual cycle, and it remains a most widely utilized natural treatment for PMS, as well as for menstrual cramps and menopausal symptoms. You will often find women's tonics that contain St. John's wort in combination with other ingredients that function similarly. Some women begin taking St. John's wort just before their PMS usually begins, while others find they must allow the herb to build up in their system, so take it all month long.

My patient Joan reported to me that "St. John's wort has definitely helped my marriage. My husband was ready to leave me because I was so miserable when I had PMS. I have been taking the St. John's wort for just over a year now, and my marriage is wonderful!" Similarly, my patient Sue reported, "It is part of the herbal 'hormone replacement' formula I take. It definitely adds an extra dimension on top of the usual herbal combination. When I had to resort to another brand without the St. John's wort, I really noticed the difference."

Q. What makes St. John's wort so effective in treating PMS and menopause?

A. The mild phytoestrogen, or plant estrogen, called beta-sitosterol in St. John's wort may account for the herb's effectiveness in treating the symptoms of anxiety and depression associated with PMS and menopause. During PMS and menopause, the level of estrogen in a woman's body is low. However, the estrogenic action of St. John's wort does not appear to cause any problems in men who take it, possibly because of beta-sitosterol's low level of activity. All phytoestrogens are mild compared with the estrogens obtained from animals or the synthetic estrogens used in hormone-replacement therapy. But studies on the effects of phytoestrogens on men have not been conducted. In more good news for men, though, there is some evidence that plant estrogens—found to one degree or another in all plants, including those in salads—help to protect men from prostate cancer.

Q. Can taking St. John's wort help attention deficit disorder?

A. Many of the symptoms of attention deficit disorder (ADD) are similar to those of anxiety and depression. While no research on the effects of St. John's wort on ADD has as yet been conducted, I have found the herb to be very useful in these cases. When treating persons afflicted with ADD, I also occasionally recommend the herbs kava and reishi mushroom. For more information on these herbs, see the "Suggested Readings" list at the back of this book.

Q. Can St. John's wort help in cases of obsessive compulsive disorder?

A. It is definitely worth a try. No research is yet available, but I have seen and heard of success in this area. Most likely, because of its serotonin-enhancing effects, St. John's wort curtails the circular thinking and obsessive worry of obsessive compulsive disorder (OCD). If it doesn't work sufficiently, I would suggest that you combine it with 5-hydroxytryptophan (5-HTP) to increase the serotonin effect. (You should be able to buy 5-HTP at most health food stores and pharmacies.) If you do this, however, you will need to watch for serotonin syndrome, which, though unlikely, can be serious. I'll explain a little more about serotonin syndrome later in this book.

Q. I took Prozac for weight loss, but it stopped working, and I didn't like the side effects anyway. Can St. John's wort help?

A. Medications similar to Prozac, called selective

serotonin reuptake inhibitors (SSRIs), enhance the effects of serotonin in the body and have been prescribed for weight loss. Unfortunately, the weight-loss effect is usually temporary. With St. John's wort, you might run into the same problem. On the other hand, since it curbs anxiety and depression, it might help with "nervous eating." Moreover, many people have reported both appetite suppression and weight loss over time with St. John's wort, and it may be a promising herb in this area.

Q. How can one herb have so many different benefits?

A. Like most plant medicines, St. John's wort is a complex substance with over two-dozen major active ingredients, each one with its own effects. These compounds work together to accomplish more than any one component could on its own. Rather than unwanted side effects, you may experience side benefits.

Of the greatest interest are the naphthodianthrones, which include hypericin and pseudohypericin; flavonol glycosides; phloroglucinols, which include hyperforin; and essential oils. The percentages in different plants vary because the chemicals in herbs are affected by the growing conditions, time of harvest, genetics of various strains, and other factors. One ingredient, hypericin, while not the main antidepressant, is used as a marker for standardization. In a recent article, researchers suggested that hyperforin may be a significant antidepressant component. As we can see, more research is needed before we can say for sure how this versatile herb works.

3.

St. John's Wort and Depression

In this chapter, I will discuss depression—what it is, how commonly it occurs, and what causes it. I will describe the signs and symptoms of the various types of depression, and explain which of these types respond best to St. John's wort. I've included case histories to illustrate my points, and describe research studies to back them up. You should realize, though, that feeling depressed is not the same as suffering from clinical depression. Left untreated, most bouts of depression last from six to thirteen months; when treated, they end in approximately three months. A diagnosis of clinical depression can be made only if a person displays a number of symptoms for a certain length of time, and only after physical causes have been ruled out. Anyone who suffers from severe symptoms of depression, such as suicidal thoughts, should seek professional help without delay.

Q. What is depression?

A. Before we look at how St. John's wort can relieve depression, we first must understand exactly what the disorder is. Clinical depression is not the brief drop in mood that comes from a bad day at the office or a fight with your spouse. Rather, it is an ongoing medical illness that can consume the life of anyone who suffers from it. Abraham Lincoln, one of many prominent people afflicted with depression, wrote: "If what I feel were equally distributed to the whole human family, there would not be one cheerful face on Earth."

There are potential causes of sadness in everyone's life, but most people manage to cope with their problems without becoming incapacitated. For example, if you lose your job, you may feel sad for a few weeks. However, if you are unable to face the world, are in tears all of the time, and feel like a failure, you would be suffering from clinical depression. In other words, the feeling you would be experiencing would be out of proportion to the external cause, and without help, you could eventually find yourself with a serious dysfunction.

Q. What is the incidence of depression?

A. A total of 18 million Americans suffer from depression. Almost one in five people can expect to suffer from some type of clinical-depressive episode in their lifetime, with women twice as prone as men. In a recent study, nearly 50 percent of the subjects between the ages of eighteen and fifty-four met the criteria for at least one of fourteen serious psychiatric illnesses. The elderly, who were not included in this particular study, have an even higher incidence of mental illness. And all evidence points to increasing rates of depression for people of all ages.

Q. Is depression something with which you are born?

A. Many diseases have a genetic, or inherited, component. So it is not surprising that research has shown depression to have a genetic component. If you are depressed, there is a 25-percent chance that a first-degree relative—a parent, child, or sibling—is also depressed. If you are not depressed, the chance is only 7 percent.

Scientists have studied the genetic predisposition toward depression in identical twins, especially twins who were reared separately due to adoption. By definition, twins share the exact same genetic material. Research has shown that if one twin becomes depressed, the other has a 40- to 70-percent chance of also becoming depressed, even if raised in a completely different environment. Meanwhile, biologically unrelated siblings raised in the same environment do not share the same incidence, nor do fraternal (nonidentical) twins or other biologically related siblings. In these cases, the correlation rates range from 0 to 13 percent. All of this proves the existence of a strong genetic component in depression.

A genetic predisposition towards illness does not mean that the illness is inevitable. It's true that you cannot change your genetic inheritance. However, you can affect the way the inheritance is expressed. For example, as we saw from the twin studies, the rate of depression does not correlate 100 percent of the time.

Q. What about the psychological contributions of environment, early experiences, and trauma to depression?

A. Research has clearly shown that not only will certain stressors cause depression as a direct response, but they may predispose the individual to future episodes of depression. Actual chemical changes occur in the brain in response to trauma, making the person more vulnerable to such future events. A lack of early love and support can also leave a mark. Many children experience abuse on numerous levels every day of their lives. According to Peter Levine in *Waking the Tiger Within*, even psychological abuse from overt bullying to the more subtle shaming, criticism, and lack of emotional support produce changes in the brain that can lead to depression.

Still more evidence of the mind-body connection is seen in the occurrence of depression in the victims of accidents, natural disasters, and wars. These victims are generally depressed, anxious, and irritable, with sleep disturbances, a variety of physical complaints, and problems maintaining jobs and relationships. Trauma of this type makes an indelible mark on the brain, and interferes with the maintenance of emotional balance.

Q. How does brain chemistry affect depression?

A. Regardless of the triggering factors, the underlying mechanism of depression is a shift in brain chemistry. The brain is made up of nerve cells, or neurons. Between the neurons are small gaps called synapses. In order for a message to pass from one neuron to its neighbor across the synapse, a chemical messenger called a neurotransmitter must be released. The presynaptic neuron—the one that is sending the message—produces the neurotransmitter, which moves toward the postsynaptic neuron on the receiving end. The neurotransmitter molecule is shaped like a key that will fit only a certain lock, called the receptor site, on the postsynaptic neuron. When the key slides into the lock, the message is received, and the receptor is either activated or inhibited, depending on its function. When there has been a shift in the brain chemistry, the key misses the lock or there are too few keys or locks.

Once its job is complete, the neurotransmitter molecule is released back into the synapse. It might return to the precursor neuron, where it can be used again, or it might remain in the synapse, along with other kinds of chemical messengers. The molecule may then continue the cycle by reconnecting with a receptor, or it may be inactivated by an enzyme called monoamine oxidase (MAO).

Q. What are some specific neurotransmitters, and what do they do?

A. One of the most important neurotransmitters is serotonin. Serotonin influences many physiological functions, including blood pressure, digestion, body temperature, and pain sensation. It also affects the circadian rhythm, which is the body's day-and-night cycle, as well as mood. Low levels of serotonin are associated with depression, obsessive thinking, anxiety, increased sensitivity to pain, emotional volatility and violent behavior, alcohol and drug abuse, PMS, carbohydrate cravings, and sleep disturbances. On the other hand, normal levels of serotonin are associated with emotional and social stability. In fact, Prozac is used to treat depression because it raises the serotonin level. However, it also has many side effects.

Other neurotransmitters that affect mood are norepinephrine and dopamine. Many antidepressants work by enhancing the effects of these neurotransmitters. St. John's wort has been shown to have similar effects, but without the side effects of these prescription medications.

Q. What can cause these variations in the neurotransmitter levels, and, conversely, can a change in mood alter the balance of our neurotransmitters?

A. Neurotransmitter levels are affected by all the factors that cause can depression. For example, genetics; environmental factors, including traumatic events; and even disappointments can cause temporary shifts in these chemicals. Nutrition also plays a part, and depression will occur if there are insufficient building blocks to make the neurotransmitters.

The building blocks of the neurotransmitters are the amino acids that come from the protein we eat.

Q. How does St. John's wort treat depression?

A. While the exact mechanism of action of St. John's wort is unclear, some are likely. St. John's wort probably affects the levels and activity of the various neurotransmitters. It was initially thought to be an inhibitor of MAO, an enzyme that breaks down the neurotransmitters. It more likely reduces the rate of how the brain cells reabsorb (that is, it inhibits the reuptake of) the antidepressant neurotransmitters—serotonin, norepinephrine, and dopamine. This leaves more neurotransmitter molecules in the synapses, thereby enhancing the activity at the receptor sites. This is similar in its action to the various antidepressants—the SSRIs such as Prozac, which affects serotonin; the tricyclics, which affect norepinephrine; and bupropion (Wellbutrin), a nontricyclic that affects dopamine. It has also been suggested that St. John's wort inhibits another chemical messenger, interleukin-6, which mediates the stress response. This gives St. John's wort an antistress effect as well.

Q. What are the symptoms of depression?

A. There are a number of symptoms that psychiatrists and psychologists look for in diagnosing depression. These symptoms include a persistent sad, anxious, or "empty" mood; pessimism or a feeling of hopelessness; a loss of interest or pleasure in the usual activities, including sex; insomnia, early-morning awakening, or excessive sleeping; feelings of agitation; decreased energy, fatigue, or a sense of being "slowed down"; low self-esteem, feelings of worthlessness, or excessive or inappropriate guilt; difficulty concentrating, remembering, or making decisions; and recurrent thoughts of death or suicide, a suicide attempt, or making a specific suicide plan.

Q. How can I tell if I'm depressed?

A. Reread the above list and take the quiz in Chapter 1. As an example, consider the words of Jana, a thirty-two-year-old dental assistant: "Here's how I know when I need help: I worry about things instead of dealing with them and then letting go. I have trouble getting to sleep. It gets hard for me to maintain my focus. I find I don't have the attention span to sit down and read books, and normally I love to read.

These symptoms can creep up on me slowly, but I have finally learned to recognize them as my early warning signs of depression. Then I increase my dosage of St. John's wort. Once you are in balance you will feel more competent to deal with everything life throws at you, you will have more patience and endurance."

Q. What about recurrent thoughts of death or suicide?

A. Between 5 and 15 percent of severely depressed people take their lives each year. While most of them keep their thoughts to themselves until they commit the act, others actually do talk about it to friends and family members. Relatives and friends need to take threats of suicide seriously, and not see them merely as attention-getting devices. Anyone who has suicidal thoughts should muster the courage to ask for help. Depression is a treatable disorder. Death is not.

Q. What are the different types of depression, and which ones can be helped by St. John's wort?

A. In conventional psychiatry, diagnoses fall into specific categories. *The Diagnostic and Statistical*

Manual of Mental Disorders is a clinical guide for mental-health professionals in which the different mental disorders are described and categorized. It was first developed in 1952 by a special committee of the American Psychiatric Association, which continues to update the manual based on current information. The classifications provide a good starting point for discussing the various types of depression. In total, there are five main categories—major depressive disorders; bipolar disorder and dysthymia; adjustment disorder with depressed mood; seasonal affective disorder (SAD); and postpartum depression.

Let's take a closer look at the five classifications, keeping in mind that they are merely guidelines, not hard-and-fast labels. Generally speaking, St. John's wort may be limited in value in the first two disorders, but very useful in treating the last three types of depression. Also important to remember is that mental disorders can result from a variety of physical disorders as well.

Q. What is a major depressive disorder?

A. This is a serious depression that interferes with normal functioning. The standard psychiatric treatments include medication and psychotherapy. While the majority of the research with St. John's wort has been done on mild to moderate depression, there has been some success in its use in major depression at higher doses—1,800 mg per day. This is an extraordinarily high dose, and you should not take it except under direct medical supervision.

Q. Can St. John's wort be used in bipolar disorder?

A. Bipolar disorder, also called manic-depressive illness, often runs in families. Far less common than the other forms of depressive disorders, it involves cycles of depression and elation (mania). Sometimes, the mood switches are dramatic and rapid, but most often, they are gradual. In the depressed phase, a bipolar person can have any or all of the symptoms of a major depressive disorder. During the manic phase, he or she may experience the symptoms of mania, which include inappropriate elation or irritability; severe insomnia; grandiose notions and poor judgment; increased speech, energy, and sexual desire; disconnected and racing thoughts; and inappropriate social behavior. A milder form of elation, called hypomania, may replace the blatantly manic phase. The hypomanic person may seem entertaining and fun, and even be creative and productive. The depressive part of the cycle, however, can still be severe and incapacitating.

Cyclothymic disorder is a milder form of bipolar

disorder. Cyclothymic individuals have moderate mood swings that can go on for years. These emotional variations are not severe enough to be considered either major depression or full mania, but they can significantly interfere with a person's life.

Despite the lack of clinical studies, St. John's wort is used regularly in Germany to treat bipolar disorder, often in combination with pharmaceuticals. More research needs to be done in this area before we can give a definite answer. I use St. John's wort in my own clinical practice, in conjunction with other supplements, including reishi mushrooms, and possibly medication, to help balance out both the depressive and manic tendencies.

Q. What is dysthymia?

A. The term "dysthymia" comes from the Greek and literally means "bad mood." Though not as severe and disabling as a major depressive disorder, dysthymia is still difficult for those suffering from it. With their mild to moderate depression, these people feel that life is mostly "just going through the motions." If you have dysthymia, you may be able to function at work or school, and possibly not even realize you're depressed. The disorder can start during childhood or later in life. In most cases, it is chronic, or long-term, in nature. Typical dysthymia consists of a depressed mood, low energy, weight gain, feelings of hopelessness, and low self-esteem.

Q. Can St. John's wort be used to treat dysthymia?

A. Research shows that dysthymia responds well to St. John's wort. Psychotherapy is also useful in these cases, and the combination may be superior to either one alone.

Q. Can St. John's wort be used for adjustment disorder?

A. St. John's wort is an excellent treatment for adjustment disorder, sometimes referred to as reactive depression. This is a temporary depression, up to six months in duration, resulting from an identifiable stressor that occurred within the preceding three months. The stressor could be the loss of a job, a divorce, or a traumatic incident such as an earthquake, accident, or fire. The stressor impairs the individual's ability to function properly in school, on the job, and in relationships. Reaction to the death of a loved one can also fall into this category. While normal bereavement time varies considerably among the different cultural groups, marked depression for longer than two months suggests a major depressive disorder.

It is important to discern whether a change in mood or personality is due primarily to an internal cause, such as a biochemical imbalance, or to an external cause, such as job stress or unemployment. Obviously, some people are more resilient than others. Early trauma often sets the stage for increased vulnerability to future traumatic events. The standard treatment can include either psychotherapy or medication, and often a combination of the two is the most effective.

Q. My doctor told me that I have seasonal affective disorder. What exactly is this disorder, and can St. John's wort help?

A. St. John's wort has been used quite successfully in the treatment of seasonal affective disorder (SAD). The lack of sunlight that occurs in autumn and winter triggers biochemical changes in the brain and leads to such symptoms as depression, impaired concentration, anxiety, marked decrease in energy and libido, and carbohydrate cravings. Also, like bears preparing to hibernate, people with SAD eat more, gain weight, and need more sleep. SAD is especially prevalent in countries at the extreme northern and southern latitudes, where there is less sunlight during the winter months. When affected individuals get their required dose of sunlight, they feel energetic and ready to get on with life.

Scientists have found light therapy—consisting of exposure to a set of full-spectrum fluorescent lights during the early morning and evening hours—to be effective. Exposure to light helps to regulate the body's production of melatonin, the hormone associated with regulating the circadian rhythm. St. John's wort can be combined with light therapy for a greater effect. In a study comparing St. John's wort to light therapy, the researchers concluded that St. John's wort is almost as effective as light therapy, with St. John's wort offering more convenient relief. In the view of herbalist Terry Willard, St. John's wort "brings light into dark places."

Q. Can St. John's wort be used for post-partum depression?

A. Postpartum depression occurs soon after childbirth and is related to a drop in hormone levels, particularly that of progesterone, which was made in large quantity by the placenta prior to birth. A combination of natural progesterone and St. John's wort is effective. However, St. John's wort is not approved for nursing mothers, so it should be used only under medical supervision, if at all. On the other hand, natural progesterone is available by prescription from compounding pharmacies, and is safe during nursing.

Lucinda, who suffered from this often improperly treated disorder, explained, "I used St. John's wort for post-partum depression and it has made a big difference in my life. I couldn't handle the side effects of the drug my doctor prescribed. Now, I can sleep better and am in more control of my emotions. It took about 2 weeks to feel a difference. It also stopped all the cramping I usually experience with my period." Lucinda's case further illustrates how St. John's wort is useful in other women's disorders, such as menstrual cramps, PMS, and even menopausal symptoms.

Q. In what cases does St. John's wort not work?

A. Anyone with symptoms of depression should receive a thorough medical examination to rule out other possible causes. Medical conditions such as thyroid disorders, anemia, hypoglycemia, chronic fatigue syndrome, and nutritional deficiencies can also cause depression.

Take Gretchen, for example. A bright, creative

hairstylist and artist, she had been depressed for a couple of weeks. "I was going home at night and crashing, not wanting to see anyone. I just wanted to sleep when I wasn't working," she said. "I had read about St. John's wort, and decided to try it for two weeks. Nothing changed. Then I remembered that I tend to be anemic, and had not taken iron for a while." When her iron was low, Gretchen would feel tired and depressed. "I went off to the health food store, bought some iron, took it daily, and within a week, was feeling back to normal."

Was this a St. John's wort failure? I don't think so. Rather, Gretchen is a great example of someone who understands her own body, looks for a recognizable pattern, and feels confident enough to take charge of her own health when necessary. If your depression is due to a deficiency of iron or some other nutrient, St. John's wort won't likely help. Your iron level can be easily checked by your doctor with an inexpensive laboratory test.

4.

Using St. John's Wort

In the United States, St. John's wort is sold without a prescription in health food stores and pharmacies. This leaves it up to you to choose the dose, form, and brand, and to be aware of any restriction in its use and any possible side effects. In this chapter, I will help you to understand the various choices, and how to select the right treatment plan for you. I will cover the precautions and side effects in a separate chapter.

In addition, for moderate depression, I recommend seeking professional help—a psychotherapist for "talk therapy" to help you deal with your life issues and to monitor your progress if you take herbs such as St. John's wort. A practitioner of natural medicine is also helpful for diagnosing and treating any underlying biochemical imbalances.

Q. What is a standardized extract, and why is it important?

A. Unlike synthetic medicines, which contain a single compound, herbs often have a variety of active ingredients. Therefore, we need to have a way of standardizing the product—that is, of manufacturing the product with consistent, measured amounts of the active ingredients per unit dose, be it capsule, tablet, or tincture. In St. John's wort, some of the active ingredients have not even been identified yet. For the longest time, experts believed that the main active ingredient was the chemical hypericin. Research, however, has indicated that this is not the case. Even so, the hypericin content is used as a convenient reference point, or marker, to create standardized extracts. It may not be the best marker, but it's the only one we have for now. So, St. John's wort products formulated to contain a specific amount of hypericin give you a consistent dosage.

If you look at the fine print on the label of a bottle of St. John's wort, you will find that most products use a 0.3-percent concentration of hypericin. This means that a 300-mg capsule of St. John's wort would contain 0.9 mg (300 mg multiplied by 0.3 percent) of hypericin. You also need to consider the amount in each dose, such as the number of drops of tincture. While other ingredients in St. John's wort may also be involved in the herb's antidepressant activity, they are likely distributed within the plant similarly to the hypericin. As a result, the hypericin standardization serves as a useful guidepost for the strength of all of the active ingredients. Extracts from as low as 0.125-percent hypericin up to 0.3 percent hypericin have yielded positive results. The original studies used the lower concentration, while most of the current studies employ the 0.3-percent concentration.

Q. Does it matter from what part of the herb a St. John's wort product is made?

A. Not all St. John's wort products utilize the same part of the herb. However, the buds, or unopened flowers, contain the highest concentrations of active ingredients, so products made exclusively from buds are generally the most potent. The opened flowers of St. John's wort contain somewhat less of the active ingredients, and the longer a flower has been open, the lower is its hypericin level. This may be true for the other active ingredients as well. The next highest source of the plant chemicals is the leaves. The remainder of the plant, including the stalk and roots, is much lower in hypericin concentration, although even these parts of the plant do have some of the active chemicals. Manufacturers generally adjust their mixtures to account for these variations.

Q. What is the recommended dose of St. John's wort?

A. As discussed above, to be sure you get a consistent amount of the active ingredients, you need to use a standardized extract. The recommended daily amount of standardized extract ranges from 0.9 mg (rounded off to 1 mg) to 2.7 mg of hypericin in divided doses. Generally, a 300-mg capsule of St. John's wort contains 0.9 mg of hypericin.

You can start by taking 300 mg of St. John's wort daily and increasing the dose gradually, upping it every few days until you reach 900 mg daily, or you can immediately start taking 900 mg daily. While the research shows that the average successful dose is 300 mg three times daily, I have known patients who required less and others who required more.

Q. What if the St. John's wort doesn't seem to work?

A. If you take 900 mg of St. John's wort daily for at least two months and still feel no improvement, you can increase the dose gradually to as high as 1,800 mg daily. There is a chance that you may not realize how much you have improved until you stop taking the herb. If this is the case, you will notice a downturn in your mood a few weeks after stopping the St. John's wort. If, on the other hand, the St. John's wort still does not work, perhaps your diagnosis should be re-evaluated. Just like some of my patients, you may need to be on antidepressant medication.

Q. What forms does St. John's wort come in?

A. St. John's wort has been available in the traditional tincture and tea forms for centuries. The most common current form of administration in the United States is the capsule, containing either fresh or dried extracts of the plants. In Europe, on the contrary, the pharmaceutical manufacturers favor the use of tablets and tinctures. You can vary these methods as long as you take the correct daily amount of active ingredient. It may take some experimentation to find the dosage that works best for you.

Q. Exactly what are a tincture and a tea, and how are they used?

A. Tinctures, which are preferred by traditional herbalists, are liquid extracts produced by soaking the crushed herb in alcohol or glycerin. The oily, active ingredients in the herb seep out into the liquid. The remaining residue is then filtered out, and the result, for St. John's wort, is a bright-red liquid that contains nearly all of the hypericin, pseudohypericin, and other active chemicals in the plant. Tinctures are normally stored in brown glass dropper bottles, tinted to help protect the active ingredients from light. The active ingredients can lose their potency when exposed to light or air.

The proper dosage of St. John's wort tincture depends on the severity of your condition, your body's ability to absorb and utilize the tincture, and the product's potency. Start with a low dose, a dropperful of tincture once or twice a day, and build up, adding another dropperful every few days, until you reach a maximum of two dropperfuls two to three times daily. With herbs, unlike synthetic medicines, there is a lot of leeway between the effective dose and the excessive. Tinctures can be mixed with water or juice to both disguise the taste and dilute the possibly irritating effects. If you wish to avoid the taste or effects of the alcohol (which are very minimal at this low concentration), put the tincture in warm water for a few minutes to allow the alcohol to evaporate.

You can also get your daily dose of St. John's wort by drinking an aromatic tea three times a day. Try to find the freshest shredded buds or flowers available, then add 2 tsp of the herb to 1 C of boiling water. Let the herb steep for 15 minutes, then drink it three times a day. If you find the taste too bitter, add some honey.

Q. What about capsules and tablets?

A. Gelatin or vegetable-based capsules filled with powdered dried herb come in a variety of sizes and strengths, so you need to read the labels to ensure that you get the proper dosage. Most capsules sold are 300 mg, so at the standardized level of 0.3-percent hypericin, each capsule contains approximately 0.9 mg of hypericin. With capsules of lower concentrations, you will need to take a higher dose (that is, more mg) to get the same amount of hypericin. If you need a lower dose, though, these capsules may be just right. More is not necessarily better. While most of the current research uses three capsules of 300 mg per day, you can adjust the dosage to your individual needs.

Tablets are powdered herb compressed into a solid pill. Again, be sure to use a standardized product that yields 0.9 to 2.7 mg of hypericin per day.

Q. How should I take St. John's wort?

A. Since St. John's wort should be taken two to three times daily, take it with breakfast, lunch, and/or dinner. While combining the herb with food does not interfere with its absorption and utilization, it does minimize any possible nausea or gastrointestinal upset. Also, taking the herb with meals makes it easier to incorporate it into your daily routine. Studies have shown that two of the main ingredients of St. John's wort have relatively long half-lives in the body. "Half-life" is the scientific term for the time it takes one-half of a substance to be broken down in the body. Hypericin has a half-life of twenty-four to forty-eight hours, and pseudohypericin has a half-life of eighteen to twenty-four hours. This means that St. John's wort has good round-the-clock activity, working even while you sleep.

Q. Can I take my entire daily dose of St. John's wort at one time?

A. While it's possible to take your entire daily dose all at once, it's always better to take smaller doses at regular intervals. This not only minimizes the potential for any side effects, but it permits a more steady level of the active chemicals in your body. This can be particularly important when you first start using the herb. Second, the antidepressant benefits of St. John's wort may be enhanced by components other than hypericin and pseudohypericin, and these other components may have shorter half-lives. So, more frequent doses may in fact be necessary to receive the full benefits. On the other hand, for convenience, you can take two doses in the morning and one with dinner. For some people, St. John's wort is stimulating and thus should be avoided close to bedtime. Others report that it helps them to fall asleep more easily. Do what works best for you.

Q. How quickly does St. John's wort work, and what should I expect?

A. Many of my patients have reported positive effects almost immediately, with a sensation of "a weight being lifted," decreased anxiety, and an enhanced ability to concentrate. As with most antidepressants, though, it may take three or four weeks before you notice a significant effect. Take St. John's wort regularly, not just when you feel down, since the antidepressant effects are cumulative. Taking larger dosages of the herb are unlikely to reduce this time lag.

Within a week to ten days, many people notice improved sleep—a better quality, fewer interruptions, and more dreaming. There may also be improvements in appetite, energy level, and physical well-being. By the second or third week, there is a reduction in emotional symptoms, with less anxiety, a more positive mood, a greater ability to handle trauma, and a sense of peace. As with any remedy, natural or synthetic, St. John's wort affects different people in different ways. Some people experience changes sooner or later than average, and some don't experience changes at all.

Many people report that they are able to handle irritants and disappointments far more easily, not getting as upset as before. Commenting on her own experience, Gayle, a thirty-five-year-old accountant, said, "I feel lighter, happier, and more energetic. Stuff just rolls off my back now. I don't have PMS any more, either."

Q. How long should I stay on St. John's wort?

A. Once its effects have stabilized, St. John's wort can be taken for as long as necessary. It has been used safely for years, with no ill effects, by many depressed patients in Europe. Halting St. John's wort generally produces no withdrawal symptoms, so you can stop and restart it as needed. Some find it better to taper off. After a few months, rather than stopping all at once, you may wish to lessen the dose gradually to assess your continued need and the dosage level at which you need it. This requires some close observation to ensure that you don't inadvertently slip back into depression.

I have had patients tell me early in treatment, with natural or synthetic medication, that they haven't noticed any positive changes, while their family members noticed marked improvements. The same is true of negative changes. So, it's a good idea to enlist a family member or friend as a co-monitor. You can also repeat the depression test, and compare your new score to the original one. Some people can tell when they are slipping, and restart their St. John's wort. It may take effect more rapidly than it did the first time, perhaps because the brain has somehow become "trained" in its response.

Q. Where can I buy St. John's wort?

A. St. John's wort is available at most health food stores and pharmacies. Pick a reputable, well-known brand that is standardized, because this will ensure that you get the same quantity of active ingredients in each dose. Even so, there are differences in quality between the brands, as evidenced by people who report doing well on St. John's wort until they change brands, despite the label's showing an equal strength of the active ingredients. When they switch back to their original brand, these people see their symptoms improve once again. Conversely, an apparent failure of St. John's wort for some individuals is turned into success when they switch brands. If you can, purchase a brand that has standardized amounts of the other ingredients as well, to be sure that you get a full complement of the antidepressant ingredients.

Look for brands that are certified organic—that is, guaranteed free of pesticides and other synthetic chemicals. Organic herbs often also have higher nutrient concentrations, yielding more healing power per flower. Wildcrafted herbs, picked and processed fresh from the woods and meadows where they grew, are an excellent source of organic herbs. However, you must know your territory before picking wild roadside "weeds." It is impossible to tell whether cattle ranchers or highway maintenance crews have sprayed a plant with herbicide, which can lead to a serious toxic reaction when ingested.

For my office, I choose supplements from a variety of manufacturers, always looking for the best quality at the lowest prices. You can also order from mail-order companies in the United States and elsewhere.

Q. Can I combine St. John's wort with other herbs and supplements?

A. Herbs that energize and balance, called adaptogens, can boost the positive effects of St. John's wort. The ginsengs—American ginseng (*Panax* *quinquefolius*), at 100 mg of standardized extract twice daily, and Siberian ginseng (*Eleutherococcus senticosus*), at 90 to 180 mg twice daily—are excellent additions.

Q. What about using kava along with St. John's wort?

A. This South Pacific herb is becoming increasingly popular for the treatment of stress, anxiety, and insomnia. At 70 mg of standardized extract taken two to three times daily, it relieves tension, both mental and physical, while enhancing alertness. At higher doses, it is an excellent nighttime sedative, producing deep, restful sleep, with no interference to REM sleep and no hangover. It has minimal side effects, is nonaddictive, and has no withdrawal symptoms. Moreover, it combines well with St. John's wort. With its earlier onset, kava is useful for handling anxiety until the antidepressant effect of St. John's wort kicks in. For resources for more information on this subject, see the "Suggested Readings" list at the back of this book.

Q. Can I mix St. John's wort with 5-hydroxytryptophan?

A. Both St. John's wort and 5-hydroxytryptophan, more commonly known as 5-HTP, increase the level of serotonin and will complement each other nicely. However, watch for signs of too much serotonin. While rare, serotonin syndrome has the following symptoms—a dangerous rise in blood-pressure, diarrhea, fever, severe anxiety, headache, muscle tension, and confusion. The first sign is often a severe, throbbing headache.

Q. What about supplementing with vitamins and minerals?

A. I always ask my patients to take a high-potency multi-vitamin-and-mineral complex. Not only are most diets quite deficient in these essential nutrients, but stress and depression deplete them further. Often, depression is a sign of deficiency, and the symptoms will improve with supplementation. The B vitamins are particularly important in depression. For resources for more information on this subject, see the "Suggested Readings" list at the back of this book.

Q. I have heard that what I eat can affect my mood. Is this true, and what can I do about it?

A. You are what you eat, and if you eat junk, your body and brain will be seriously compromised. Here are some basic dietary guidelines: To begin with, eat lots of fresh, organic fruits and vegetables. These will provide you with vitamins, minerals, antioxidants, and other nutrients. Eat seeds, nuts, and whole grains, which haven't had all of their nutrients stripped away. Avoid processed foods—that is, foods in boxes or cans—as much as possible. Not only are these foods devoid of "life force," but they contain dangerous additives. For example, the artificial sweetener aspartame is known to be toxic to the brain. I have seen many people whose severe anxiety and even bizarre behavior cleared up when they stopped drinking aspartame-containing diet soft drinks.

Also, eliminate (as best you can) white flour and sugar, and other empty-calorie foods. Reduce your overall fat intake. Avoid saturated fats and fried foods. Instead, eat foods rich in the essential fatty acids, specifically flax, soy, pumpkin-seed, and walnut oils, and cold-water fish such as salmon and mackerel. Avoid sources of caffeine, such as coffee, tea, and cola drinks. Limit your alcohol consumption to one drink (4 oz of wine) per day. Drink at least eight 8-oz glasses of pure water a day. Considering that our bodies are 65-percent water, we must not ignore this life-giving element.

Q. I notice that I feel better when I exercise, and get depressed when I stop doing it regularly. Why?

A. Exercise enhances all of your metabolic processes by increasing the circulation of blood and oxygen to all the parts of your body, including your brain. Also, exercise prompts your body to release greater amounts of powerful, mood-elevating endorphins, which produce the sensation known as runner's high. There have been over 100 clinical studies done examining the link between endorphins and exercise, proving that exercise can be as effective an antidepressant as medication and traditional psychotherapy. You do not have to be a seasoned athlete to benefit from exercise, either, although the more intensely you exercise, the more endorphins your body produces.

5.

Precautions and Side Effects

In this chapter, I will discuss the precautions you should consider before taking St. John's wort, and the side effects for which you should watch. The incidence of side effects is very low, especially when compared to those of the prescription medications. I will explain whether or not St. John's wort can be combined with alcohol, and if there are any foods or medicines to avoid while taking it. Remember, too, that everybody is different, and what is good for one person may not be good for another. Therefore, you need to learn to trust your own responses. Most people do very well with St. John's wort, experiencing no side effects at all.

Q. How does St. John's wort compare with other medications regarding side effects?

A. The low incidence of side effects with St. John's wort gives it a clear advantage over the other available medications for depression. While Prozac and the other antidepressants may be effective at treating depression 60 to 80 percent of the time, many patients stop taking them because of the side effects. The side effects of these medications include nausea, headaches, anxiety, insomnia, drowsiness, diarrhea, dry mouth, loss of appetite, sweating, tremors, loss of short-term memory, and rashes. As if all of this weren't bad enough, most antidepressants also reduce the sex drive and may interfere with sexual functioning. Ironically, these antidepressant medications can give you something to really be depressed about!

Q. What side effects have been reported for St. John's wort?

A. Even when side effects do occur with St. John's wort, they are milder than those produced by synthetic medications. Some patients taking St. John's wort complain of dry mouth, dizziness, gastrointestinal symptoms, fatigue, and increased sensitivity to sunlight. St. John's wort also occasionally produces lightheadedness or dizziness associated with standing up suddenly, called "postural hypotension." If you experience this, get up slowly to avoid falling and injuring yourself.

Gastrointestinal symptoms are the most common side effects of St. John's wort and include nausea, loss of appetite, abdominal pains, and diarrhea. There are some simple solutions for this problem: Take your doses with meals, so that food can buffer the irritating effects. If you use an alcohol-based tincture, switch to one with a glycerin base. In addition, lower the overall dose, or simply divide your daily dose into smaller portions. I have also seen side effects stop when patients switch brands. Allergic reactions including skin rashes and itching have also occurred. Many people find that they are able to reduce their daily dose and eliminate the side effects while still receiving the antidepressant benefits of the herb. Of course, all side effects stop when intake is stopped.

Q. What has research shown regarding the side effects of St. John's wort?

A. A European drug-monitoring study looked at the experiences of 3,250 patients treated with St. John's wort. It found that only 2.4 percent of the patients reported any side effects at all, a rather remarkable finding when you consider that Prozac produces side effects at least ten times more frequently, and that even placebos (supposedly inert pills) produce side effects. Doses of St. John's wort up to thirty-five times the standard dose have been given to human volunteers with only minor side effects. No deaths from St. John's wort in humans have ever been reported.

Q. Can you become addicted to St. John's wort, and are there any problems when you stop taking it?

A. Unlike most of the psychoactive drugs, St. John's wort is not addictive, and there are no withdrawal symptoms upon stopping it.

Q. Can you drink alcohol while taking St. John's wort?

A. Unlike antidepressants and many other medications, St. John's wort produces no adverse effects when mixed with alcohol. This is not to suggest that you actually have a St. John's wort cocktail, or even that you drink at all. However, having an occasional drink while taking St. John's wort is not a problem.

Q. Is it true that you have to stay out of the sun when taking St. John's wort?

A. Phototoxicity, or increased sensitivity to the sun, was considered in the past to be a major concern with St. John's wort. However, for the vast majority of individuals, there is very little chance of ever developing this condition. The FDA noted that light-haired cattle and sheep, after consuming great quantities of the plant while grazing in the sun, developed serious sunburn, and many even died. This led the FDA to put St. John's wort on its unsafe list, where it remained for many years. However, a 1993 human study found that the usual therapeutic doses used for depression are thirty to fifty times below the level at which phototoxicity occurs.

The only people who are likely to experience phototoxicity are persons with acquired immunodeficiency syndrome (AIDS) who take extremely high amounts of the herb for its antiviral properties and are then exposed to the sun. This condition is most likely to affect fair-skinned individuals, who have less natural pigmentation and protection from the sun's damaging rays. To be cautious, use sunscreen if you take high doses of St. John's wort, and avoid major sun exposures, especially if you are fair-skinned or sun-sensitive. Also, do not graze naked in the sun on large quantities of St. John's wort, especially if you are a light-skinned sheep.

Q. I found that after a week on St. John's wort, I felt more anxious. I lowered my dose, and my anxiety cleared up. Is this common?

A. I have seen a few cases of anxiety from St. John's wort. Since it is likely related to the onset of treatment and the associated biochemical changes in the brain, the anxiety should disappear after the first few weeks, as it does with the SSRI medications. The best course of action is to reduce your dosage until your anxiety resolves. If it persists, stop taking the herb completely; it may not be the right treatment for you. In one study, anxiety occurred only in one out of 400 persons (0.26 percent). A far higher rate of 9 percent has been reported with SSRIs such as Prozac, particularly at the start of treatment.

Q. Is there anyone who should not take St. John's wort?

A. If you have a medical condition or take a medication, be sure to speak with your doctor before beginning St. John's wort. While the herb is much safer than the prescription antidepressants, these factors may make you more sensitive to its effects, and you may need a lower dosage. In any case, even with a natural medicine like St. John's wort, it is always wise to use the lowest effective dose. This is especially true if you have a liver or kidney disease, since these two organs are involved in the processing of all medicines.

While there is no evidence that St. John's wort can produce birth defects, I advise pregnant and nursing women not to use it, at least until research to the contrary is available. In general, children under the age of twelve should also not be given St. John's wort because we have no specific research on its effect on kids. Of course, children are given a variety of antidepressants, and common sense would say that St. John's wort is a safe substitute. However, until more data is available, it should be administered to children with care and only under appropriate medical supervision. The dose should be adjusted to the child's lighter weight, considering that the adult dosages are for a 150-lb person. I also recommend that St. John's wort, as all medications, even nonprescription, be kept out of the reach of small children.

Q. I have heard that there is a long list of medicines and foods to avoid when taking St. John's wort. Is this true?

A. It was initially recommended that people taking St. John's wort avoid foods containing the amino acid tyramine, as well as MAO-inhibiting (MAOI) medicines such as 5-HTP and L-dopa, for fear of causing an unsafe rise in blood pressure. However, newer research has shown that this side effect occurs in test-tube experiments, but not in people. In fact, St. John's wort likely works through other mechanisms, such as by inhibiting the uptake of serotonin and other neurotransmitters.

Q. Can St. John's wort raise my blood pressure?

A. Hundreds of thousands of people with high blood pressure in Germany use St. John's wort without any problems. Nevertheless, I have seen increases in blood pressure from the use of the herb, even when other medications are not used. There is no research information available on this, so use your own judgment. Often, the first sign of elevated blood pressure is a persistent, severe pounding headache, particularly in the back of the head or over the temples, that becomes worse when lying down. While not common, if this occurs, have your blood pressure checked immediately and discontinue your use of St. John's wort.

Q. Do I need a doctor's supervision to take St. John's wort?

A. In the best of all possible worlds, medical help would be easily and cheaply available, with a choice of appropriate herbal medicines. Obviously, this is not always the case, and you must do what is practical for you. If you are not under medical care, I urge you to watch carefully for side effects.

If you take St. John's wort for longer than a month and/or for moderate depression, you should contact your doctor. Have your blood pressure and heart rate checked every month, and have your blood count, liver enzymes, and kidney function checked every four to five months. You should also monitor your mood, alertness, sleep patterns, and energy levels, plus retake the quiz in Chapter 1 to check your progress. If a side effect is serious or troubling in any way, you should immediately stop using the St. John's wort until you get a medical diagnosis of your condition. What may seem to be a minor side effect could actually be a sign of a much more serious physical or mental disorder that needs to be addressed.

6.

Other Uses of
St. John's Wort

A holistic view of medicine does not separate illnesses into two neat stacks—physical ailments and mental ailments. To begin with, many physical disorders can lead to depression, and depression can lead to physical illness. In addition, the mind-body continuum has common influences, and imbalances can occur throughout the system. In this context, St. John's wort is an excellent antidepressant that also boasts a remarkable range of other healing properties. It has antiviral, anti-inflammatory, and antibacterial effects. Its sedative and pain reducing effects make it useful for treating neuralgia, fibromyalgia, sciatica, and rheumatic pain. It also may have some anticancer properties (though it is not a cure). As a lotion, St. John's wort will speed the healing of wounds, bruises, varicose veins, mild burns, and sunburn. In this chapter, I will discuss some of St. John's wort's other uses.

Q. Can St. John's wort be used to treat chronic viral infections?

A. St. John's wort has been shown to have significant antiviral activity, although in dosages much higher than those required to treat depression. Experiments, both in test tubes and in animals, have indicated that two of the active chemicals in the plant, hypericin and pseudohypericin, are clearly effective against a number of viruses, including flu, herpes, hepatitis C, and Epstein-Barr. The Epstein-Barr virus is associated with infectious mononucleosis and chronic fatigue syndrome. St. John's wort has also been investigated as a treatment for AIDS. Compared with other antiviral medications, St. John's wort has very few side effects, although it can cause some phototoxicity when administered in very high doses.

Q. What about using St. John's wort for chronic fatigue syndrome and fibromyalgia?

A. I have had dramatic successes in treating these difficult conditions with St. John's wort. Not only is St. John's wort's antiviral activity effective against chronic fatigue syndrome, but its anti-inflammatory action relieves the body aches and tenderness of fibromyalgia. It also eases the depression, fatigue, and anxiety of the two conditions.

Renata, who was depressed, achy from fibromyalgia, and constantly exhausted from chronic fatigue syndrome, exemplifies what St. John's wort can do for these disorders. When Renata consulted a specialist at a major university medical center, she was told simply that she should rest. Then, a clerk in a health food store suggested that Renata take St. John's wort at a dose of 300 mg three times daily. Within a few weeks, Renata's depression lifted and her energy began to return. By six weeks, she was not only free of symptoms, but noticed that she did not suffer her regular herpes flare-up with her menstrual period. A year later, Renata is still taking St. John's wort and remains symptom-free. Her case is a great illustration of St. John's wort's multiple functions. Her experience is particularly remarkable considering the usual difficulties in treating both chronic fatigue syndrome and herpes.

Q. Can St. John's wort be used for HIV and AIDS?

A. At New York University, Drs. Meruelo and Lavie researched the use of hypericin in fighting human immunodeficiency virus (HIV), the virus associated with AIDS. They found that in mice, hypericin not only inactivated the virus, but also shielded the membranes (walls) of healthy cells from attack. No other current antiviral drug is able to do this. It is also possible that hypericin, if added to donated blood, may protect transfusion recipients from becoming infected with HIV, though more research is needed to confirm this.

Q. Is St. John's wort still used to treat infections, wounds, and burns, as it was in the past?

A. Several studies have confirmed the traditional use of St. John's wort in wound healing. The plant has antibiotic chemicals in its flowers and leaves. One German study showed that using an ointment containing the herb reduced healing time dramatically and resulted in less scarring. First-degree burns healed within forty-eight hours, and third-degree burns healed three times faster than normal and without the usual formation of scar tissue.

A friend of mine verified St. John's wort's healing powers through personal experience. When her four-year-old son accidentally scalded his hand with boiling water, she immediately applied St. John's wort oil to the burn site. The pain ceased, and the boy stopped crying. The redness cleared in a few days, leaving none of the blistering or scarring that generally follows such a burn.

St. John's wort acts against a wide variety of bacteria. In one study, it was found to be more effective than the antibiotic sulfanilamide against the *Staphylococcus* (staph) bacteria responsible for many hospital infections. In addition, the bacteria that causes tuberculosis, the fungus *Candida*, and the gastrointestinal parasite *Shigella* all have responded to St. John's wort. These findings are particularly important because of the increasing incidence of antibiotic-resistant strains of bacteria. While you should never use St. John's wort in place of appropriately prescribed antibiotics, you can use it to enhance your immunity so that you are better able to fight infections.

Q. What do St. John's wort's anti-inflammatory and immune-enhancing actions do?

A. Until the advent of antibiotics, battlefield medics used St. John's wort ointments. This was because, as Russian researchers recently discovered, this complex herb contains substances that both stimulate and suppress immunity. Because of this, St. John's wort has the ability to boost the immune system to fight infection, while at the same time damping the immune processes that promote inflammation. Substances that can perform this balancing act are called tonics, or adaptogens. Synthetic medicines have only one active ingredient, so they simply can't manage such a harmonious balancing of the body's immune response.

Q. How about treating sciatica with St. John's wort?

A. St. John's wort has historically been used for treating nerve injuries and spinal-cord pain and injuries, including crushed and pinched nerves. One of my patients, Josh, said, "I have been using St. John's wort for my sciatica [nerve-root pain that radiates from the back down the leg], and it's the best relief I've ever had—better than aspirin or ibuprofen. I can now exercise and play basketball, with no setbacks."

7.

The Scientific Basis of St. John's Wort

When patients ask about the uses and benefits of herbs and other natural remedies, most conventional doctors say, "There's no proof," simply because they don't know about natural therapies and the research that validates them. In this chapter, I will describe the scientific research that has been conducted with St. John's wort. In addition, I will take a brief look at the future that awaits this wonderful herb.

Q. Why do we need research to prove that St. John's wort works?

A. Research studies are the backbone of conventional medicine. They provide us with a wealth of valuable information in all fields, including human biology and the health sciences. But scientific research is not unbiased research. It is complicated by factors that determine which therapies receive funding and which do not. Research is costly, running into the millions, and most natural products do not have major funding behind them. In Europe—where many herbs are classified with other pharmaceutical products, prescribed by doctors, and covered by national health plans—it's a different story. Because herbal medicine is accepted in Europe as a legitimate form of therapy, the pharmaceutical companies there have the financial incentive to do the necessary research.

Q. Why are drugs better researched than herbs in the United States?

A. In North America, a pharmaceutical company will bear the cost of a research study only if it can patent the new product that results from the research. The worldwide antidepressant market, for example, is worth an estimated $6 billion annually. Natural products such as herbs can't be patented, and discoveries made about them become public domain, so the manufacturers of these products witness insufficient returns on their investments.

As a result of the pharmaceutical companies' huge investments in their products, and because of their collaborations with medical schools for research purposes, much of the information taught to doctors in medical school and beyond comes from the pharmaceutical companies themselves. However, the demand is growing in North America for a more natural approach to medicine, including the use of products such as herbs. Therefore, it is likely that the American pharmaceutical industry will follow the European lead and create refined extracts, which can be patented. Unfortunately, this will involve focusing on the so-called active ingredients and removing the "extra" substances, which are what actually make herbs the powerful healers they are. On the other hand, since the current herbal research is pointing in the direction of "whole" extracts, this approach may instead dominate.

There is still a great deal that needs to be discussed regarding these topics, and we will have to watch carefully that herbs, including St. John's wort, are not made prescription-only items, resulting in restriction of their use.

Q. What has the research shown about St. John's wort?

A. Much of the available research on St. John's wort was conducted in Europe and most of the results were published in German, thus causing the research to miss being noticed by American scientists. Then, in 1996, a significant and extensive review article on St. John's wort was published in the *British Medical*

Journal. This study caused the scientific and medical communities to sit up and take notice, since the *British Medical Journal* is world renowned for its high standards. The authors did a meta-analysis—that is, they analyzed twenty-three randomized clinical trials looking for overall conclusions. Fifteen of the studies compared the herb with a placebo, and eight compared it with conventional antidepressants, in a total of 1,757 outpatients.

The meta-analysis found that St. John's wort did slightly better than the antidepressants in eliciting a positive response—63.9 percent of the subjects found relief with St. John's wort and 58.5 percent found relief with the antidepressants. However, only 0.8 percent of the subjects taking the herb dropped out of the study because of side effects, while 3.0 percent of the subjects taking an antidepressant ended their participation early. In summary, when compared with a placebo for treating mild to moderate depression, St. John's wort worked far better, with a 60- to 80-percent success rate, which is equal to that of the standard antidepressants, but with far fewer side effects.

Q. Are there any problems or questions regarding the European research?

A. While the European results look promising in relation to the use of St. John's wort as an antidepressant, the information has some limitations, and further research is needed.

First, all of the studies reviewed were of short duration, lasting just four to eight weeks. Most antidepressants "kick in" after a few weeks, but may take longer than eight weeks to build up to their maximum effectiveness in certain individuals.

Second, the doses of the antidepressants used in the control groups were relatively low. Thus, we don't know how well St. John's wort works compared to high doses of these medications.

Third, St. John's wort has not been compared to the SSRIs, such as Prozac, Zoloft, or Paxil; to the MAOIs, such as Nardil and Parnate; or to Effexor (venlafaxine hydrochloride), which functions like the tricyclics but without the side effects, inhibiting serotonin reuptake, while at the same time boosting the norepinephrine level. St. John's wort has been compared in humans only to the tricyclic antidepressants (specifically amitriptyline, imipramine, and maprotiline), and in rats and mice to the tricyclic antidepressants, plus a nontricyclic called bupropion (Wellbutrin). It has been found to be similar to these antidepressants in effectiveness. However, the results of animal studies don't necessarily reflect what the effects on humans would be.

Fourth, there are language and cultural differences between the United States and Germany that may affect the interpretation of the German results by American researchers.

In any case, the United States has a bias regarding "foreign" standards, and the American medical establishment is more likely to accept American-based research results.

Q. Is any American-based research being conducted with St. John's wort?

A. The National Institute of Mental Health, together with the National Institutes of Health Office of Alternative Medicine and the Office of Dietary Supplements, has begun the first American-based, large-scale clinical trial on the use of St. John's wort for clinical depression. This $4.3-million, three-year study is being coordinated by Jonathan Davidson, MD, of Duke University Medical Center. Using a well-defined sample of adequate size and duration, the study will assess the herb's effectiveness, safety, and side effects with long-term use, as well as the users' risk of relapse.

The study will include 336 patients with major depression, as defined by the fourth edition of the *Diagnostic and Statistical Manual of Mental Disorders*.

The subjects will be assigned randomly to one of three treatment options for an eight-week trial. One-third of the participants will be given a specific dose of St. John's wort, another third will be given a placebo, and the remaining third with be given Zoloft, an SSRI commonly prescribed for depression. The acute controlled phase of the study will last for eight weeks and will be followed by a four-month follow-up of the patients who responded to treatment. The study will take about three years to complete, with the data analysis to be completed some months later.

Q. What can we look forward to as far as the acceptance of St. John's wort by mainstream medicine is concerned?

A. The public has been expressing a growing interest in herbal products to treat mental and other illnesses, and wants scientific evidence to support their use. Conventional medicine has responded by beginning to explore the potential contributions of these products to health. In a 1998 study by John Astin, Ph.D., of Stanford University, published in the May issue of the respected *Journal of the American Medical Association*, 40 percent of the respondents said that they had used some form of alternative health care during the preceding year. This was up from 33 percent in a 1993 study published in the *New England Journal of Medicine*. Moreover, in the 1998 study, anxiety was tied at 31 percent as the second most frequently cited health problem treated with alternative therapies.

Conclusion

You now know how St. John's wort works, as well as when and how to use it for depression. I have discussed the research with it and the clinical evidence of its effectiveness, and described how it compares favorably with the synthetic antidepressants. People with mild to moderate depression can be successfully treated with St. John's wort without having to sacrifice their quality of life or health. We find in this herb an unusual combination of safety, effectiveness, a broad range of positive effects, a lack of side effects, and low cost. The extensive European research with St. John's wort was positive, and the National Institute of Mental Health is now conducting its own $4.3-million study, comparing St. John's wort both to a placebo and to known pharmaceutical antidepressants.

The popularity of St. John's wort has brought a renewed recognition and acceptance of herbal medicine by average people who are looking beyond conventional medicine for solutions to their health problems. My professional preference is that individuals not self-diagnose or self-treat. However, there are economic realities that make professional help unavailable to many people. In any case, self-treatment with St. John's wort is often all that is needed. We are part of nature, and natural substances are much more compatible with our human biology than synthetics could ever be. Our dependence on technological medicine, including pharmaceuticals, has not yielded increased freedom from disease. Rising health costs are also pointing toward the use of these far less costly products.

This is an exciting time to be a physician, with many new possibilities for healing opening up every day. I believe that most doctors are motivated and curious to find the best, least harmful approaches for helping their patients. I therefore recommend that you take this book to your doctor to help teach him or her about the benefits of herbal medicine in general and of St. John's wort in particular. Fortunately, the patients who seek complementary care tend to be those who are most likely to take responsibility for their own healing and least likely to expect the doctor to do or know it all. Sharing this knowledge can help you, your doctor, and your doctor's other patients.

Let us use St. John's wort as a bridge between conventional and alternative therapies, and continue to open up the vast realm of natural treatments. This expanded approach can lead us full circle to an increased appreciation of our natural resources. Sustaining what we have and renewing what we have destroyed is our only hope for the future—of humanity, of the planet, and of all living beings.

Glossary

Amino acids. The breakdown products of protein that form many components of the body including the neurotransmitters, which affect mood.

Biochemical. Related to the chemistry of the body or of other living things.

Genetic. Linked to the genes that carry the chemical blueprint with which we are born. Genes are passed from parent to child, and can include a tendency to depression and other disorders. Many diseases have a genetic component.

Half-life. A scientific term referring to the time it takes for one-half of a substance to be degraded in the body.

Marker. A convenient reference point when creating standardized extracts. For St. John's wort, the marker is the hypericin content. Using a marker ensures that the product has a specific amount of activity in every dosage unit.

Neuron. A nerve cell in the brain and other parts of the nervous system.

Neurotransmitters. The chemical messengers of the brain. Serotonin, norepinephrine, and dopamine are the best known, and a deficiency of any one produces depression. Another neurotransmitter, gamma-aminobutyric acid (GABA), is related to both anxiety and depression.

Phototoxicity. A severe reaction from exposure to the sun that was considered in the past to be a serious side effect of St. John's wort. However, for the vast majority of individuals, there is very little chance of ever developing this condition.

Serotonin. An important neurotransmitter, thought to be enhanced by the use of St. John's wort.

Synapse. Refers to the space between the neurons in which the neurotransmitters circulate.

References

Astin JA, "Why patients use alternative medicine," *Journal of the American Medical Association*, 20 May 1998.

Blumenthal Mark, Gruenwald J, et al., *The German Commission E Monographs*, English translation (Austin, TX: American Botanical Council, 1998).

Hansgen KD, "Multicenter double-blind study examining the antidepressant effectiveness of the hypericum extract LI 160," *Journal of Geriatric Psychiatry and Neurology* 7 (1994):S15–S18.

Harrer G, "Clinical investigation of the antidepressant effectiveness of hypericum," *Journal of Geriatric Psychiatry and Neurology* 7 (1994):S6–S8.

Linde K, Ramirez G, Mulrow CD, Pauls A, Weidenhammer W, Melchart D, "St. John's wort for depression: an overview and meta-analysis of randomized clinical trials," *British Medical Journal* 313 (1996):253–258.

Meruelo D, et al., "Therapeutic agents with dramatic antiretroviral activity and little toxicity at effective doses," *Proceedings of the National Academy of Sciences USA* 85 (1988):5230–5234.

Suzuki O, et al., "Inhibition of monoamine oxidase by hypericin," *Planta Medica* 43 (1984):272–274.

Thiede HM, "Inhibition of MAO and COMT by hypericum extracts and hypericin," *Journal of Geriatric Psychiatry and Neurology* 7 (1994):S54–S56.

Thiele B, Brink I, Ploch M, "Modulation of cytokine expression by hypericum extract," *Journal of Geriatric Psychiatry and Neurology* 7 (1994):S60–S62.

Woelk H, Burkard G, Grunwald J, "Benefits and risks of the hypericum extract LI 160: drug monitoring study with 3250 patients," *Journal of Geriatric Psychiatry and Neurology* 7 (1994):S34–S38.

Suggested Readings

Breggin, P. *Talking Back to Prozac*. New York: St. Martin's Paperback, 1995.

Cass, H. *Kava: Nature's Answer to Stress, Anxiety, and Insomnia*. Rocklin, CA: Prima Publishing, 1998.

Cass, H. *St. John's Wort: Nature's Blues Buster*. Garden City Park, NY: Avery Publishing Group, 1998.

Lee, J. *What Your Doctor May Not Tell You About Menopause*. New York: Warner Books, 1996.

Levine, P. *Waking the Tiger Within*. Berkeley, CA: North Atlantic Books, 1997.

Murray, M, and Pizzorno, J. *Encyclopedia of Natural Medicine*. Rocklin, CA: Prima Publishing, 1994.

Nelson, J. *Sacred Sorrows*. New York: Tarcher/Putnam, 1996.

Pert, C. *Molecules of Emotion*. New York: Scribner, 1997.

Shapiro, F, and Forrest, MS. *EMDR*. New York: Basic Books, 1997.

Slagle, P. *The Way Up From Down. New York:* Random House, 1987.

Index